No More Moles, Warts, or Skin Tags™

How I Safely Removed Moles, Warts, and Skin Tags for Life

By Chris Gibson

UMM
UNIVERSAL MARKETING
MEDIA, INC.

Published by Universal Marketing Media, Inc.

No More Moles, Warts, or Skin Tags™

How I Safely Removed Moles, Warts, and Skin Tags for Life

By Chris Gibson

UNIVERSAL MARKETING MEDIA, INC.

Published By Universal Marketing Media, Inc. in association with Chris Gibson.

Universal Marketing Media, Inc. is a publishing and marketing company. 1216 Raymilton Rd., Polk, PA 16342, U.S.A.

The Universal Marketing Media logo is a trademark of Universal Marketing Media, Inc. Visit our website at http://www.universalmarketingmedia.com. Printed in the United States of America

Chris Gibson
http://www.molewartremoval.com
chrisg@molewartremoval.com

Gibson, Chris
No more moles, warts, or skin tags / How I safely removed moles, warts, and skin tags for life / Chris Gibson.
p. cm.
Includes bibliographical references and index.
ISBN 0-9764272-1-4
1. Health - Healing – United States. 2. Health - Healing – Canada. I. Gibson, Chris. II. Title.

Website design by teknekconsulting.com.
Book design by Fritz Conroy / TekNek Consulting, Inc
Production coordinated by Universal Marketing Media, Inc

OBLIGATORY LEGAL NOTICE:

While all attempts have been made to verify information provided in this publication, neither the Author nor the Publisher assumes any responsibility for errors, omissions, or contrary interpretation of the subject matter herein. Any perceived slights of specific persons, peoples, or organizations are unintentional. The Author neither makes nor attempts to make any diagnosis or cure or prevent any disease.

This publication is an information product, and is not intended for use as a source of legal, accounting, or tax advice. Information contained herein may be subject to varying national, state, and/or local laws or regulations. All users are advised to retain the services of competent professionals for legal, accounting, or tax advice.

The purchaser or reader of this publication assumes responsibility for the use of these materials and information, including adherence to all applicable laws and regulations, federal, state, and local, governing professional licensing, business practices, advertising, and all other aspects of doing business in the United States or any other jurisdiction in the world. No guarantees of income are made. Publisher reserves the right to make changes. If you cannot accept these terms, kindly return the product. The Author and Publisher assume no responsibility or liability whatsoever on behalf of any purchaser or reader of these materials.

Dedication

This book is dedicated to mole, wart and skin tag sufferers around the globe. But most of all it is dedicated to you, our reader - the mole, wart, and skin tag free customer of tomorrow.

Acknowledgements

Thanks to my many clients for the contributions they have made to this work. Without their thirst for information and without their faith, I would not have been challenged to dig so deeply, to probe so many crannies, and to look beyond the easy answers to find a truly natural solution. Because of you, the information in this book has evolved to what it is today.

To the entire staff of Universal Marketing Media, Inc., I say a hearty, "Thank you." You are a unique group of caring and competent people. Thanks for being who and what you are. Without you I could have never have completed this book on time.

Additionally, I wish to acknowledge the countless individuals, organizations and companies who gave so generously of their time and ideas. ***No More Moles, Warts, or Skin Tags***™ developed not only from my own experiences, but also from those of many others. Sincerest thanks to everyone!

About the Author

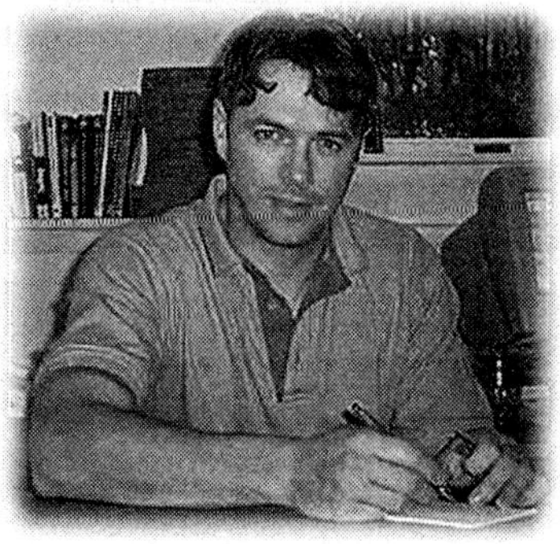

As part of a rewarding career in natural healthcare, Chris Gibson has written several books on alternative healing and wellness. When Chris began his career as an author, however, his first book was about a completely different subject: Advertising.

The huge success of his advertising book spurred him on to new and more challenging projects. In subsequent books, Chris began to share his knowledge of effective "all-natural, drugless therapies."

For many years Chris battled his moles and warts, enduring countless visits to his doctors, numerous surgical procedures, and costly prescription drug therapies and over-the-counter products. Like many suffering from moles and warts, these standard methods didn't work for Chris.

Determined to overcome his difficult condition, Chris researched the problem thoroughly and finally happened on a safe, effective, and natural remedy. This method quickly removes moles, warts and skin tags regardless of how long you have had them, and does so without the use of drugs or harsh creams. The all-natural methods described in Chris's book attacks the moles, warts, and skin tags at their source, making them disappear quickly.

Like thousands of Chris's satisfied customers, including many celebrities and dignitaries, you will be truly amazed by the results.

Chris lives on his ranch near Pittsburgh, Pennsylvania. When he is not writing, Chris spends time in his organic gardens, travels, and trains his two Labrador retrievers, Tiki and Max.

Other Titles Published by Universal Marketing Media

Acne Free in 3 Days™: How I Cured My Acne Condition in 3 Days by Chris Gibson. This best seller on natural acne cures is popular worldwide and has helped thousands end their struggle with acne once and for all. In this book, Chris Gibson shows you how he cured his acne in three days. You can do the same, without expensive prescriptions or over-the-counter products. Get your own copy and enjoy clearer skin in a matter of days! Click on the link below to read more about this book.

http://www.acnefreein3days.com

How I Permanently and Safely Cured My Athlete's Foot and Jock Itch in Under 7 Days by Scott Young. Embarrassed and discomforted by his athlete's foot and jock itch, the author confronted them against all odds. Scott developed an all-natural, unbelievably fast and permanent method for curing these extremely painful conditions. By following his proven method, you can eradicate them permanently. Click on the link below to read more about this book. Get your copy today!

http://www.cureyourathletesfoot.com

Have you ever been awakened by your partner while sleeping? Have your ever woken up feeling like you did not get a good night's rest? If so, you know that snoring is a serious problem. Though there are literally hundreds of different snoring aids, devices, and pills available on the market, thousands of people still suffer from snoring. Juan Walker was one of those people until he decided to try a different approach. In the book, ***How I Naturally Cured My Snoring Condition for Life***, Juan shows you how he easily and permanently stopped snoring. You can do the same. Get your copy today by clicking on the link below.

http://www.stopyoursnoringnow.com

With over 5 hip surgeries, numerous complications, and the early onset of osteoarthritis, Nancy MacGranahan knows what the pain of arthritis is all about. In her book, ***Arthritis Free for Life***, Nancy shares her story of how she naturally ended the pain in one month. Nancy provides you with a veritable fountain of pain relief that has left the medical profession completely amazed. Her method does not involve a change in diet or impossible exercise regimens. This is a method for real people. It works for the thousands of clients who have read Nancy's book and it will work for you too. Click on the link below to read more about this innovative treatment!

http://www.arthritisfreeforlife.com

Weight Loss by the Numbers. Everyone knows being overweight is the number one health problem in America. Though increasing numbers of Americans are overweight, they don't need to be. This effective and thoughtful plan for weight loss provides results for individuals of all ages. The author, Chris Gibson, shares with you how he was able to lose twenty-eight pounds and three pants sizes in only three weeks. You can do the same without using any worthless diet plans, dangerous pills or expensive supplements. A must read for anyone struggling to lose weight and keep it off. Get your own copy today!

http://www.weightlossbythenumbers.com

How I Naturally Cured My Allergy Condition for Life is an inspiring book by Gary Young. A registered nurse, Gary explains how he spent years battling his own life-threatening allergy condition, and how he was able to get rid of them in five days. Using his natural treatment, you too can put an end to many types of allergies, including dust mites, hay fever, pet allergies, sinusitis, pollens and molds, hives, insect bites and stings. Click on the link below to read more about this book and to get your own copy today!

http://www.allergyfreein5days.com

How I Permanently and Safely Cured My Cold Sores for Life. Anyone who has suffered with cold sores knows how embarrassing, frustrating, and painful they can be. The author, Grace Melgarejo, knows your pain because she dealt with cold sores for over twelve years. In her book, she shares her painful story but explains how you can easily cure your cold sores or herpes simplex one virus in only three days by using an all-natural method. This method has worked for the thousands of clients who have read Grace's book and it will work for you too! Get your own copy today by clicking on the link below.

http://www.coldsorefreedomin3days.com

How I Banished My Bad Breath and Gum Disease for Life. If you are one of the millions of people who struggle with mouth, gum or breath problems, then this is the book for you. The methods outlined in this book do what sprays, mints and mouthwashes cannot—they attack these difficult conditions at their source. Included in the book is a widely available but little known cure for even the most stubborn oral health issues. These natural remedies will banish your bad breath and gum disease for good. The methods are scientifically proven, easy to follow and 100% effective. Click on the link below to read more about this book and to get your own copy today!

http://www.banishbadbreath.com

How I Naturally and Safely Cured My Asthma Condition for Life. If you are one of the millions of people who struggle everyday to breathe, this is the book for you. The methods outlined in this book do what drug therapies, over-the-counter products and useless devices cannot. The methods will help you to banish your asthma permanently. These techniques do more than contain the symptoms; they actually attack asthma at its source. Click on the link below to read more about this book and to get your own copy today!

http://www.asthmafreeforlife.com

Table of Contents

Introduction

Life is full of unexpected events that touch our hearts, broaden our perspectives, and change how we live on this earth. How we see ourselves during these events, that is, our self-esteem, matters more than we realize.

If your mind is filled with doubt, these precious moments will escape you; a chance for joy will be lost. Simply put, if you are not able to enjoy the special moments in life, you are not living.

Though no one is perfect, we are all perfectly unique. We have special features and personalities that not only make us different, they make us who we are.

This is one of the things that make life so wonderful. Everyone is different and everyone is special in some way. The sooner we understand this, the sooner we can stop worrying about what other people think about us.

There is an old saying, "We must learn to accept that people are individuals - warts and all."

Well if you are like me, accepting people as they are is not a problem. But we should not accept warts (genital warts included), moles or skin tags when we do not have to do so, especially if they are painful or in a place that is just painful to look at.

My name is Chris Gibson and I have had my own personal experience with warts and moles - just like 90% of the population. As an avid gardener who worked in the landscaping business for over five years, my skin has been exposed to all kinds of elements and soils, and spent hundreds of hours under the sun.

Much of the soil in gardens contains bacteria and viruses that cause warts. So, from time to time, I have had to deal with them on my hands and feet.

For all of you who have followed the traditional path to get rid of moles, warts or skin tags as I once did, I am sure you know all too well how stubborn they can be. You also know that standard treatments rarely get rid of them permanently.

This is the main reason why I am sharing my personal experiences with you today. I want to provide you with the only ALL-NATURAL to remove warts, moles and skin tags.

These methods apply nothing harmful or harsh to your skin, but something natural that you will watch in amazement over a period of just a few days. For most people, these techniques cause the moles, warts or skin tags to simply dry up and fall away.

For others, they will dissolve and simply wither away. Either way, you will be rid of these pesky things for life!

The information you are about to use is very simple and easy to follow. I wanted to make it easy for anyone to use, so don't be put off by the simplicity.

In fact, these techniques work so well that I recommend you get started today. But before beginning, I suggest you read through the entire book and the frequently asked questions before following any of the steps.

Doing so will help you learn the process in its entirety. The better you understand the steps you need to take, the less time it will take you to do them.

Besides the book, all you will need are the easy to find ingredients. With them in hand, you will be on your way to a wart, mole and skin tag free body.

"I am not a doctor and I am not intending to treat or cure any disease; I'm simply sharing my personal experience with moles, warts and skin tags, and what I found that worked for me and works for so many others."

My Story

I have had plenty of experience with warts and moles. At 41, I have seen almost everything that a body can do.

Fortunately, I am extremely healthy and take great care of myself. As a result, I look much younger than my real age. Part of my secret is keeping the occasional skin problem in check.

My first experience with a wart was on my writing hand. It grew right where my pen hit my hand. Writer's block took on a whole new meaning!

About a week later, two more appeared on near my left handthumb. I was pretty freaked out, but I did the first thing almost everyone does...

I went down to the drugstore and bought some liquid salycilic acid wart remover. With great confidence and my "Wart-B-Gone" in hand, I went home to cure my problem.

“Here today - Gone tomorrow”, said the box. I thought to myself, “This has to work!” It did ... almost!

I carefully followed the directions of the wart remover. It was supposed to kill the wart and virus, but because I smeared on too much I ended up killing a lot more.

For nearly a month I applied the elixir and watched as layer after layer of skin peeled away, sometimes painfully. The worst part was that I did not know when the warts would finally disappear.

I stared at my hands day and night, wondering if I was ever going to rid myself of these annoying things. Not to mention, my writing suffered because the pain in my hands made it almost unbearable.

Six weeks into using the treatment, however, there was a huge change. Finally, the affected area started to look much better and new skin began to grow. The pain I encountered while writing began to dissipate and I actually enjoyed holding a pen again.

But just when I though my life would get back to normal, the bottom dropped out from under me again.

One morning, about a week after I stopped using the treatment, I woke up in complete shock and dismay. The same three little spots of warts were coming back!

It wasn't as if they just showed up a week later, they really took their time. It almost seemed as if the warts were smiling back, "We are not going anywhere," they said, "no matter what you do!"

Well, they came back all right and this time they were larger than before. Even worse, they now bled unpredictably.

This caught me by surprise and frightened me; so instead of continuing with my search for a successful removal process, I threw in the towel. As you can probably imagine, I went to see my doctor.

AMA Wart Removal Strategies

Before I continue with my story, I want to describe the three most popular surgical strategies for removing warts. They will give you an idea of what treatments you can expect when seeing your doctor.

Electro-Surgery or Electrocautery:

Electrosurgery or Electrocautery is a treatment used to kill many different types of warts. The process of removal begins with the application of a current and/or the cutting of the warts by an experienced doctor.

After giving appropriate anesthesia, the doctor uses an electrified or heated needle, blade, or wire to remove the wart growth. This treatment of warts is typically used when the warts are small in size and number.

The major drawback of this wart treatment is the high risk of scarring or disfigurement of the treated area. Pain is also a concern.

The procedure produces potentially infectious smoke. Below are before and after pictures of the process:

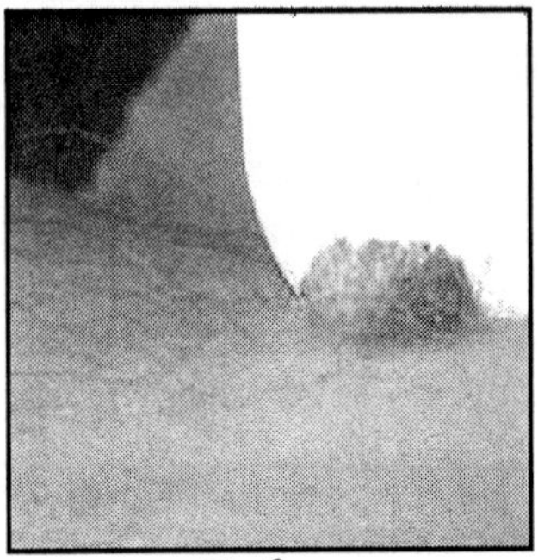
Before

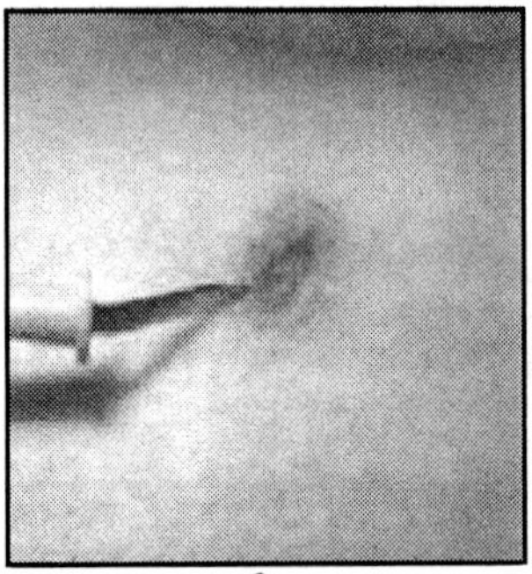
After

Laser Therapy:

Laser therapy uses a beam of high intensity laser light that is applied carefully on the affected area to destroy the warts. This procedure requires local, regional, or general anesthesia, depending on the severity of the warts.

Laser therapy is effective when used on warts that are more extensive in number and larger. It is also effective on warts in places that are difficult to reach with other treatments.

Treatment for warts with laser therapy causes less adjacent tissue injury than in Electrosurgery or Electrocautery. However, the drawbacks of laser therapy are serious and cause most people not to follow through with the treatment.

Problems associated with laser therapy include: its relative costliness, longer healing time, scarring, less availability, hospital visits, and the potentially infectious plume during the procedure.

Cryosurgery or Cryotherapy:

Cryosurgery or Cryotherapy is the most commonly used surgical strategy for wart removal. This treatment is applicable for all types of warts, including the external and internal genital areas.

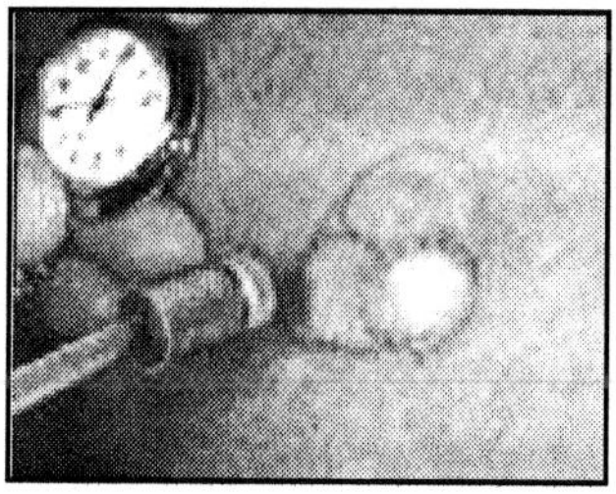

The affected areas are frozen with the liquid nitrogen (a very cold gas). The gas is applied with a cryoprobe directly onto the warts. This freezes the wart tissue and forms a blister, which later separates from the affected skin.

Cryosurgery can be very uncomfortable, but it usually isn't too painful. The freezing sometimes numbs the surrounding skin tissue.

When your doctor places the instrument on your skin, it will feel like an ice cube. Afterward, you may feel a burning sensation as your skin thaws out.

It often takes several visits and/or months before all the warts can be cleared. Healing after cryosurgery usually lasts from 1-2 months. Cryosurgery has been known to leave scars, but most people escape the process with little damage to their skin.

Also, after the area has healed, the treated skin may be a bit lighter in color than the skin around it. The drawbacks of Cryosurgery are: cost of treatment, visits to the doctor, pain associated with the procedure, and risk of scarring.

Important Note: Surgical treatments can be painful, may lead to blood loss, and need proper care to reduce the risk of infections during the period of healing.

Disclaimer: This information is not meant to be a substitute for professional medical advice. It is always best to consult with a physician about serious health concerns. This information is in no way intended to diagnose illnesses or offer remedies.

My Story Continues...

As I sat in my doctor's office waiting to hear his opinion about whether or not these were warts and not some kind of skin cancer, I wondered if he was going to excise them *in toto*, that is, cut them out of me completely.

I wondered how painful that would be and if it would keep me from getting my work done.

"Good News," he said, as he entered the room. "These are just common warts caused by a virus under your dermis (skin), and we can take care of all them today."

"They won't bother you anymore, after we treat them." I was very excited at the possibility of getting rid of my warts the same day, but then I asked the dreaded question.

"So how are you going to treat them?"

As his Nurse Practioner (a real nurse) entered the room carrying a canister that looked like a small propane torch, my doctor explained, "We are going to super freeze your skin in those areas. That will kill the wart and some surrounding skin but once it heals, you'll be good to go!"

Before I knew it, they were freezing the 3 warts. If I thought the store bought wart remover was painful...the pain from this procedure was ten times worse.

In fact, the freeze was the same as burning the skin. I now had 3 black pulsating spots that were hurting really bad. I could see I was not going to be able to write or do anything significant with that hand for some time.

My doctor was unfazed. He said it would take about a month for the three frozen spots to heal. I will spare you the gross details of how skin heals from a freeze burn.

If you have ever seen what frostbite can do to a person, this was quite similar. Suffice it to say, it was not a pretty sight! It was painful and frustrating to watch it heal.

Once again, those same three warts healed. “Wart free,” I went back about my business.

This time, things were great for about three months, but right before Christmas – here they were again – starting to come back! I felt sick to my stomach. I could not—I would not—go through that freezer-burn process again.

I thought, "There HAS to be another way”. Thank God there is!

The Natural ANSWER!

To explain how I found this removal method for warts, moles and skin tags, I have to digress a bit. In my teenage years and into early adulthood, I had some severe bouts with acne.

I waged a long battle over ten years, but I was finally able to cure my acne. Now that is another story for another day, but in the search to cure my acne, in bits and pieces I found the information on how to remove naturally warts, moles and skin tags.

At the time, I paid little attention to this information because I had no problems with warts, moles, or skin tags. However, I jotted down a few notes just in case I bumped into someone that had wart, mole, or skin tag problems.

It was only in my frustration with conventional treatments of warts that I remembered it my earlier research.

I went back through my notes, and fortunately I had saved these valuable techniques. I eagerly got the information I needed, and immediately began the simple process.

After testing it and finding it to be fairly effective, I added a couple of more steps to see if I could increase the effectiveness of the removal method. To my surprise, after making those changes the method was now ready to be used.

To remove my warts, I first took a needle and scratched the surface of each of the warts. Then, I took an emery board and scraped the area, taking it from rough to very smooth. The scratching and scraping enabled the next step to work more efficiently.

Next, I combined castor oil (usually thought of as a laxative), and a little baking soda to make a paste. I applied the mixture three times daily and covered the warts with a band-aid. The band-aid kept the paste moist.

The paste is most effective when it is wet. This is why you apply the mixture three times a day, which keeps it at its optimal consistency.

The first time I applied the paste, I felt a tingling or stinging sensation that let me know the paste was penetrating the wart. This part of the process is crucial. If you do not feel such a sensation, you need to scratch the surface of the wart again.

After Day One, I continued applying the mixture three times daily and kept it covered with a band-aid. I intended to keep this regimen up, until the warts disappeared permanently.

My notes told me the healing process would take anywhere from 3 days to 3 weeks. However, I figured it would take a month or longer for me, since the warts had been so stubborn.

I knew these warts were very resistant; they had already grown back after two conventional removal methods! But for some reason, this time I had a great feeling they were not going to survive.

I followed the plan precisely and patiently. I did not skip a day and I did not lose hope or faith. At the end of the process, the results were amazing!

15 Years of Mole, Wart, and Skin Tag Removal Results

At the end of the first week, I noticed the warts were looking much smaller. For moles, on the other hand, the opposite is true: the moles will start to get bigger. Still, I wondered if it was just because I had kept them moist.

I continued to apply the mixture three times a day. On the morning of the 11th day, as I peeled off the first band-aid on my right hand, the wart came off and fell right to the floor!

The skin around the area where the wart used to be was also perfect. I just couldn't believe it! The excitement grew as I peeled away each band-aid. The other two warts also fell off!

All of the warts that had tormented my hands for so long were gone and to this day, some 15 years later, they have never returned! After such success with removing my warts, I asked a family member to try this on a mole and skin tag she wanted to remove.

Although the process seemed a bit time consuming at first, she decided to give it a full go. As she soon found out, the process does not take much time each day. Like me, she was 100% happy with her results.

The mole fell off in less than 2 weeks and the skin tag only took 8 days. From these results, it was clear that the process works the same for moles, skin tags and warts. It just had to be tweaked a little for getting rid of genital warts.

As I have learned over the years, it is truly wonderful to have great, unmarred skin. It really affects the way you live your life from top to bottom. The more confidence you have in yourself, the more you will be able to accomplish in life.

This is why I believe the following information is so important. It will literally change your life, just as it has changed mine!

In the next sections, you will expand your knowledge base about moles, warts, skin tags, and genital warts. Each section provides a wealth of information so you can learn more about what is attached to your skin and what steps you need to follow to remove them.

Just follow the instructions and you too can permanently remove any mole, wart (genital warts included) or skin tag. The specific steps to remove moles, warts and skin tags vary slightly.

Different instructions are offered below. The total cost of the supplies is usually between than $5.00 - $10.00! Good Luck and God Bless!

All About Warts

What is a wart?

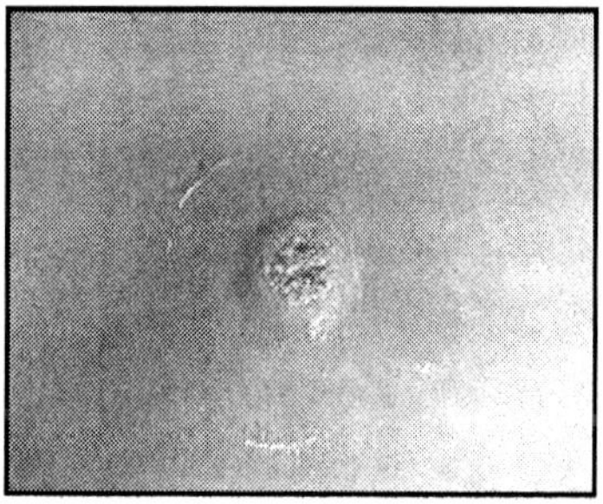

A wart is an intra epidermal or skin tumor caused by a variety of viruses. It comprises a small, circumscribed tumor of the outer or horny layer of the skin. The many varieties of warts are named by their appearance or location.

They can be level with or elevated from the surrounding skin and are usually firm. Mainly caused by the human papilloma virus, they vary in size and may be accompanied by pain, especially if they occur in the feet.

The human papilloma virus belongs to the family of viruses that causes warts. It has also been implicated as a possible cause of genital cancers and, more recently, cancers and other abnormal growths of the eye.

Types of Warts

Common Warts (Verruca Vulgaris)

These usually grow on the fingers and on the backs of hands (see picture on previous page).

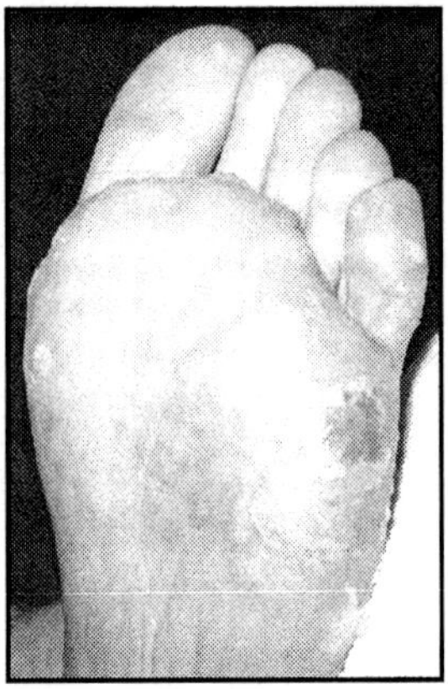

Foot Warts (Verruca Plantaris)

These are usually on the soles or the plantar area of the feet and are called plantar warts.

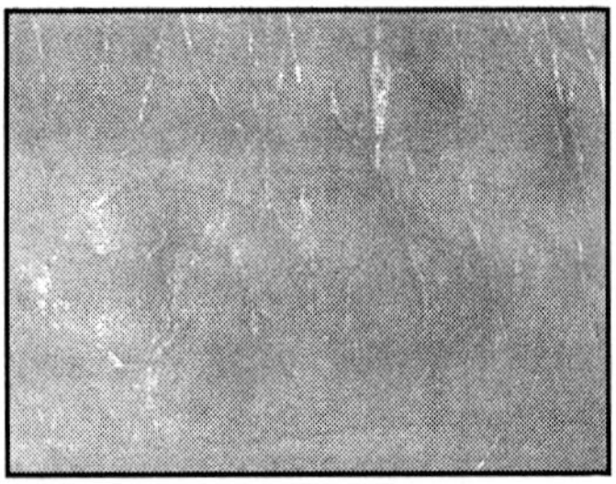

Flat Warts

These are smaller and smoother than other warts and tend to grow in large numbers, up to 20 to 100 at a time. They can grow anywhere. Among children, they usually found on the face. In adults, they are often found in the chin area in men and on the legs in women.

Genital Warts

These grow on the genitals and rectal area.

Mosaic Warts

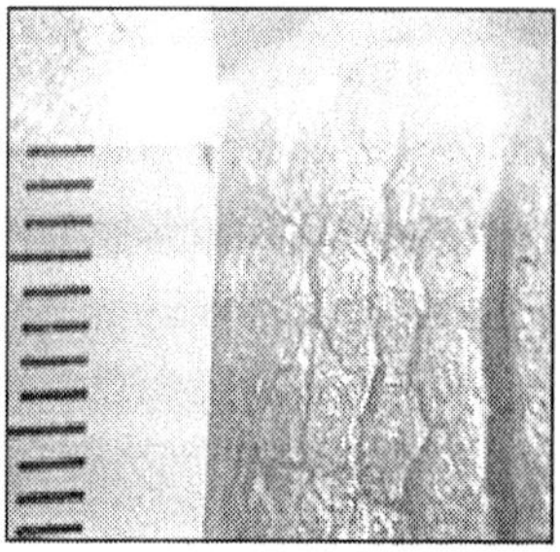

Mosaic warts are so named because of the large number of warts that appear in a contiguous pattern. The Mater (mother) wart will present itself in the center, surrounded by small, satellite lesions.

Characteristics of Warts

Contagious and Autoinculable

Warts may be passed from one person to another through skin contact. It is also possible to get warts by using objects previously touched by a person who has warts.

Genital warts can be transmitted to another person during sexual intercourse. Among women, warts can grow undetected on the cervix or inside the vagina. Carriers of genital warts may infect their sexual partner without knowing it.

Capable of Spreading and Forming Daughter Warts

Warts are known to spread to other parts of the body, and more importantly, to other people. In a few cases, they have also been known to heal by themselves. However, treatment is important not only to prevent a spreading, but to eliminate the wart(s) completely.

Infectious in Origin

As with other viral infections, warts are highly contagious. As such, one can "self-spread" these lesions.

Plantar warts commonly begin in areas where skin is traumatized. One can also get them from communal areas such as locker rooms, bathrooms, and hotel rooms.

To minimize the spread of warts to others in such settings, the use of disinfectants and sandals is encouraged.

Post-Treatment Problems with Surgeries and Other Products

High Recurrence Rate of Warts

Depending on the treatment method, different recurrence rates have been recorded. A common treatment currently used in the United States is a self-applied, 5% imiquimod cream that stimulates the immune system to fight off the virus and lesions. It has a recurrence rate of about 13-19%.

Sometimes large warts are surgically removed under local anesthesia. This has a recurrence rate of about 21%. In a study using self-applied podofilox gel, the cure rate was approximately 51%, but the recurrence rate was only about 10%.

For cryosurgery, the recurrence rate is quite high at 73%.

With my methods, in contrast, the recurrence rate of warts is a very low 3-5%.

How will I remove them?

The application process of removing a wart targets the center of the wart. When using the method, make sure the center to of the wart is sufficiently scratched for the mixture to penetrate properly.

Supplies:

The following is a list of things you will need to do the wart removal method:

1. *Small Bottle of Castor Oil*

Castor oil is widely available at grocery and drug stores. It can also be found online by searching for Castor Oil in any major search engine. There is only one kind of Castor Oil.

2. *Baking Soda (Bicarbonate of Soda)*

Baking soda is widely available at grocery and drug stores.

3. *Sterile Stainless Needle*

Sterile stainless needles are widely available at grocery and drug stores.

4. *Emery Board*

Emery boards are widely available at grocery and drug stores.

5. Band-aids

Band-aids are widely available at grocery and drug stores.

The All-Natural Method to Remove Warts:

1. Clean wart(s) with soap and water. Pat dry, but leave the wart(s) damp.

2. Scratch the entire wart(s) surface with a sterile, stainless needle. Concentrate on the wart's center or base. Use the emery board to scratch and rough up the entire surface of the wart(s). Scratching should be hard enough so that when the mixture is applied it will penetrate the wart's surface. If you have performed this step properly, a slight stinging sensation should occur when you apply the mixture.

3. Mix a teaspoon of Castor Oil with just enough baking soda to make a thin paste, not cake-like or crumbly. If the mixture takes on such a consistency, you will need to add more oil. **A new paste should be used each time you apply the mixture to your wart(s).**

4. Rub a small amount into the wart(s) until it is partially absorbed (this will take approximately 1 or 2 minutes). Make sure you apply enough so the areas you have scratched are covered completely.

5. After the initial application, apply a little more of the mixture over the top and cover with a band-aid.

6. Repeat steps one, three, four, and five, 3 three times a day: Once in the morning, once in the afternoon, and once again right before you go to bed. **You will not have to scratch the surface of the wart after the first time.**

7. Be Patient! It usually takes from 3 days to 3 weeks for the wart(s) to fall out. However, since everyone's body is different, the process may take longer. For this reason keep doing this process until the wart has fallen off completely.

Important Notes:

Scratching is the most important part of the process, since it allows the mixture to penetrate to the core of the wart(s)! If you can't use both hands, you may need another person to help you with that step.

Certain types of wart(s) are very hard. It usually helps to soak them in warm soapy water for 20-30 minutes before scratching. If necessary, simply scratch harder to penetrate the outer layer.

If a slight stinging sensation is not felt, the mixture has not penetrated the wart(s) and the application may not work properly. Scratch deeper and reapply.
Prior to using the method, calluses covering wart(s) should be softened and removed by immersing them in warm to hot water for 15-20 minutes

Treated wart(s) should be covered at all times when the mixture is applied. Be careful not to disturb or remove the band-aid, because premature removal can slow the healing process. The wart(s) will usually fall off anywhere between 3 days to 3 weeks, though some individuals may take as long as six weeks.

Redness on the skin around the treated wart(s) is a natural occurrence, and indicates the healing is progressing. Such discoloration quickly disappears.

Pink or red tissue is normal after the wart falls off. Normally, the pinkness fades as the tissue becomes environmentally conditioned. Skin tones normally balance out within 15 days, although some people may require several weeks for skin tones to return to normal.

Precautions:

The castor oil and baking soda mixture is for external use only. If the mixture gets into the eyes, flush thoroughly with water. If unusual discomfort arises, consult a physician.

It worked! What can I do to make sure they don't come back?

Vitamin A

Vitamin A in lotions and creams is vital for healthy skin and a great complexion. Though little known, Vitamin A in a topical lotion helps remedy rough, dry skin for people suffering from psoriasis.

Boosting Your Immune System

As with other viruses, boosting your immune system helps to ensure that the warts don't return. There are literally hundreds of products available to boost your immune system. You may want to check with your physician about which would be right for you.

All About Moles

What is a mole?

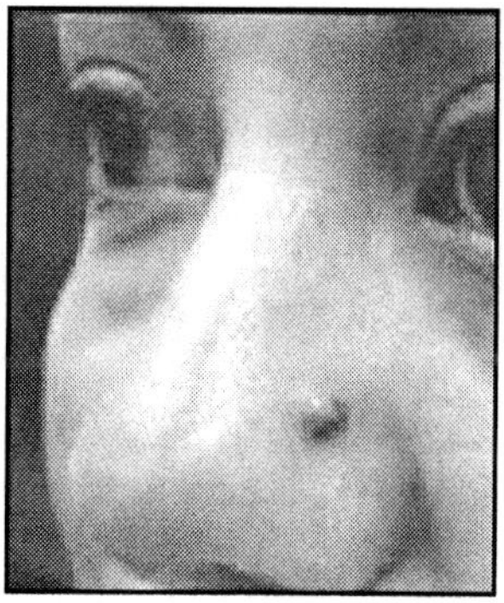

Moles (nevi) are a nevucellular skin occurrence located in the skin's various layers. Perceived by most people as a dark brown spot, moles actually have a wide range of appearance.

Though moles are sometimes considered fashionable and even called "beauty marks," not all moles are beautiful.

They can be very unsightly, such as when they protrude from the skin. Some moles may contain dark hair and they may even be dangerous.

Moles can appear anywhere on the skin and they are usually brown in color. They can also take a variety of sizes and shapes. They sometimes darken with exposure to the sun, during the teen years, and during pregnancy.

Most moles appear during the first 20 years of a person's life, although some may not appear until much later in life. Sun exposure may darken existing moles and increase their number. Some moles, however, disappear when an individual reaches about 70 years of age.

AMA Mole Removal Surgical Strategy

Surgical removal is the most common treatment for skin moles. While most skin moles do not cause serious problems, a cancerous skin mole that is left untreated is likely to increase in size. Depending on the type of cancer, such moles may spread to other parts of the body.

I offer this information about the surgical removal of skin moles so you can understand clearly what these invasive procedures entail. Such knowledge will highlight the differences between 100% natural mole removal described in this book and other methods.

The Procedure:

Removing a mole is usually a quick and straightforward procedure that does not need an overnight stay in hospital. The treatment may be available at a GP surgery or a hospital, where it is performed as an outpatient or day case.

The procedure is usually performed with a local anesthetic. In a smaller number of cases, a general anesthetic is applied prior to the procedure. The choice of anesthetic will depend upon the size and location of the mole.

A local anesthetic usually involves one or two injections to the skin around the mole. After a few minutes, the injections numb the area completely so that the mole can be removed, ideally without pain or discomfort. The local anesthetic lasts approximately two hours.

The technique for removing the mole depends on a variety of factors, such as the moles size and location. Typically, the mole is "shaved" down with a surgical blade, or is cut out (excised). The resulting wound site may require sutures (stitches).

Here is a graphic representation of a mole being removed and then sutured:

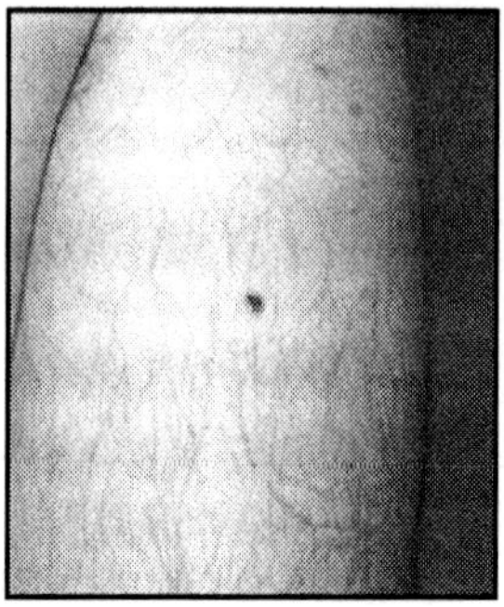

1

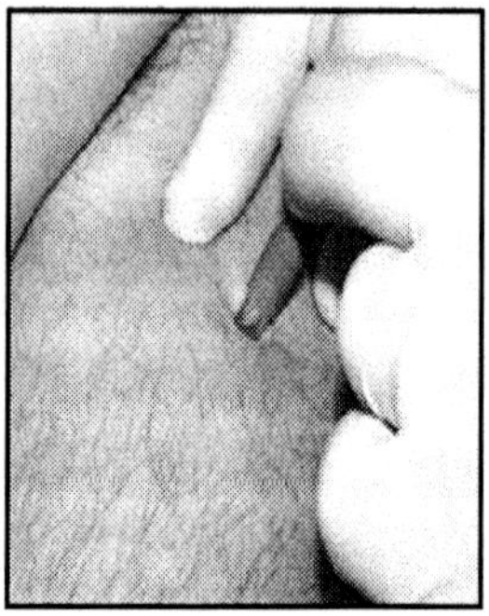

2

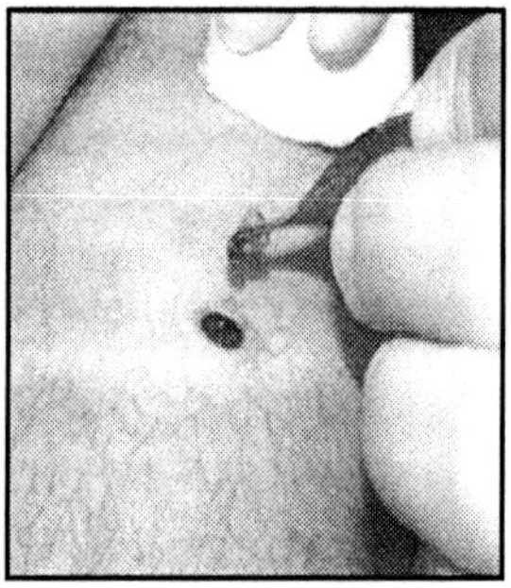

3

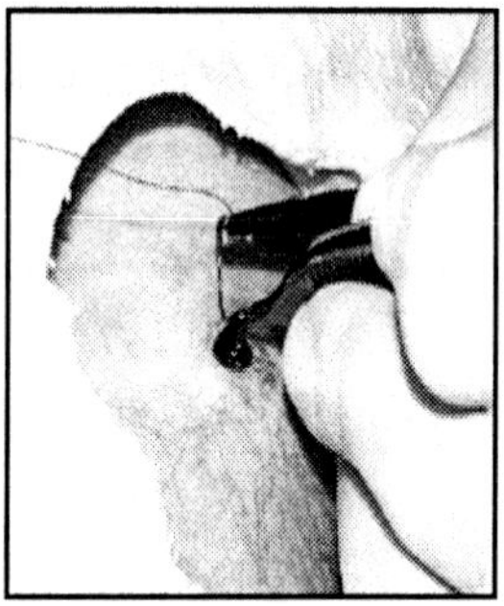

4

What to Expect Afterwards:

After having a rest and some light refreshment, most patients are able to return home within two hours of the procedure. It is sensible for people who have this operation to have someone drive them home.

Special care will need to be taken not to bump or knock the affected area, especially because the skin around the operation site will be numb for a couple of hours. As the local anesthetic wears off, the area where the mole was removed may feel sore.

Painkillers such as ibuprofen or paracetamol will help with localized pain, and should be taken as directed on the packet or by your doctor.

If the wound has a dressing, it will need to be left in place for 48 hours. Some wounds do not require dressings, since they heal more quickly when left uncovered and allowed to breathe.

Most surgical wounds do not require any special bathing and simply need to be kept clean and dry. However, when a mole has been removed from the face, make-up should be avoided in the wound area until the stitches have been removed.

The doctor or nurse will be able to give further advice and a follow-up appointment will be made if necessary. A GP or district nurse may remove any stitches five to ten days after the procedure. Dissolvable stitches disappear in around seven to ten days.

After removal of a skin mole, the wound generally heals fairly quickly. However, contact your doctor or hospital if the wound:

- Becomes more painful.
- Looks red, inflamed or swollen.
- Smells unpleasant.
- Leaks any sort of liquid.

Any of these symptoms may be a sign of infection and should be investigated by your doctor.

Healing:

The scar will go through three phases during the healing process. For the first three months, the scar is likely to be red and slightly elevated. It will then fade to pink for several months, and finally, *about a year after surgery*, the scar should closely match the rest of your skin and be flat and soft, thought it might remain a somewhat pale.

Deciding to Have the Procedure:

Having a skin mole removed is generally a very safe surgical procedure. However, in order to give informed consent for treatment, potential patients need to be aware of the possible side effects and the risk of complications.

Side Effects:

Side effects are the unwanted but usually temporary effects of a successful treatment. For this operation, they are likely to include:

- Numbness caused by the local anesthetic.
- Some pain, swelling and/or bruising around the operation site.

The operation will leave a scar. Depending on the location of the skin mole and how much healthy skin has to be removed, post-operative scars may be noticeable to others. Most patients' scars will heal normally.

Complications:

Complications are unexpected problems that can occur during or after the procedure. Most people are not affected. The most common complications of any surgery are excessive bleeding during or soon after the operation, infection, and unexpected reactions to anesthesia.

A small percentage of people have an inherited tendency to form scars that are unusually red and raised. Such scars are known as keloids and are more common in people with darker skin.

Other complications for this operation are uncommon, but their risk may increase depending on the nature of the skin mole, the exact type of operation, and other factors such as the person's general health.

For example, people who smoke or who have diabetes are at higher risk of having wounds that heal slowly. The doctor will be able to explain how these types of risks apply to each patient.

Important Note:

Surgical treatments can be painful, may lead to blood loss, and need proper care to reduce the risk of infections during the period of healing.

Disclaimer:

This information is not meant to be a substitute for professional medical advice. It is always best to consult with a physician about serious health concerns. This information is in no way intended to diagnose illnesses or offer remedies.

Types of Moles

Junctional Moles

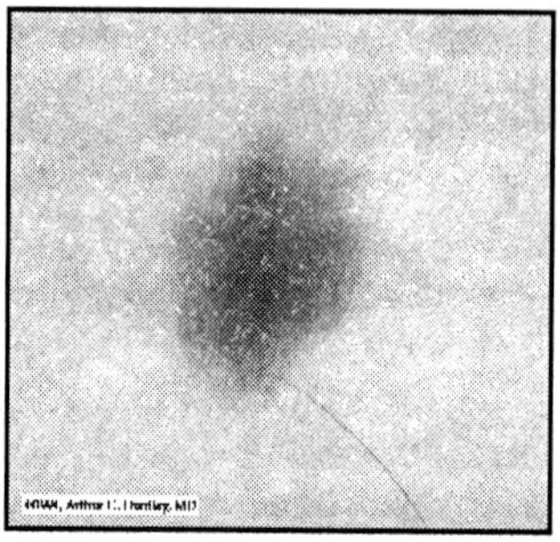

Usually brown in color and may be either flat or slightly raised.

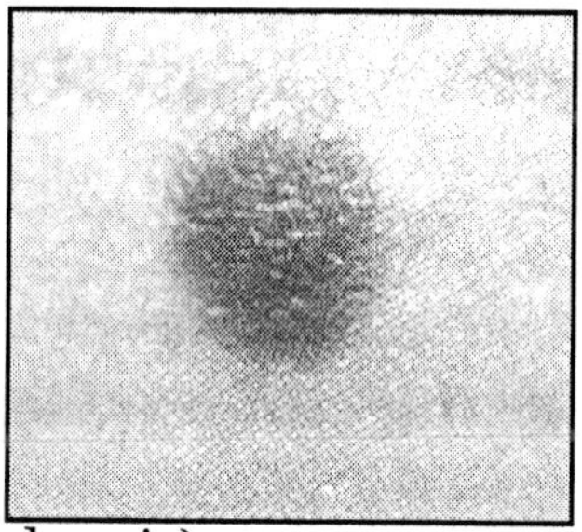

Compound Moles

Slightly raised, range in color from tan to dark brown, and involve pigment-producing cells (melanocytes) in both the upper and lower layers of the skin (epidermis and dermis).

Dermal Moles

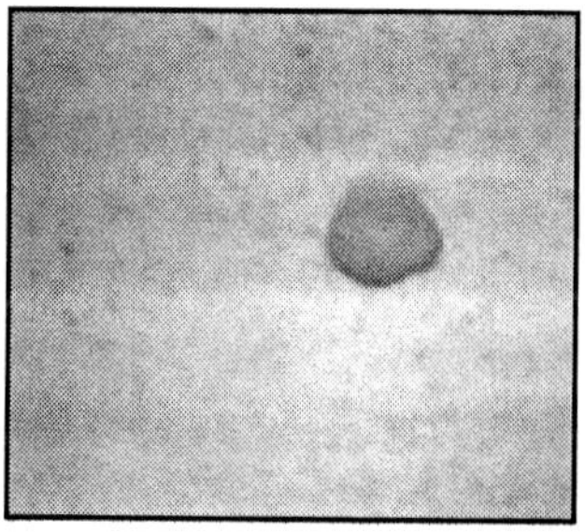

Range from flesh-color to brown, are elevated, and may contain hairs. They are most commonly found on the upper body.

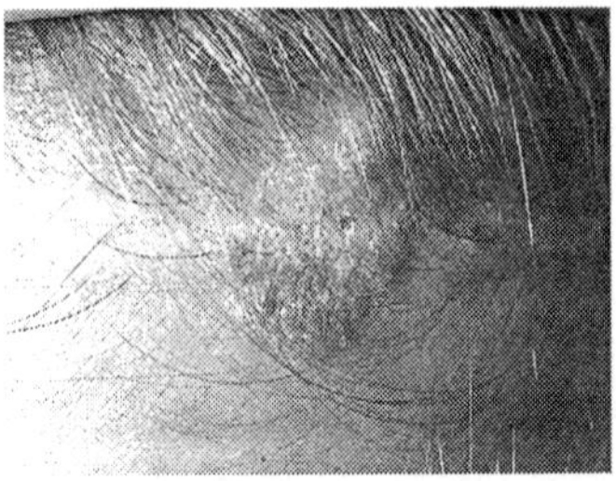

Sebaceous Moles

Produced by over-active oil glands and are yellow and rough-textured.

Blue Moles

Slightly raised, colored by pigment deep within the skin, and most common on the head, neck, and arms of women.

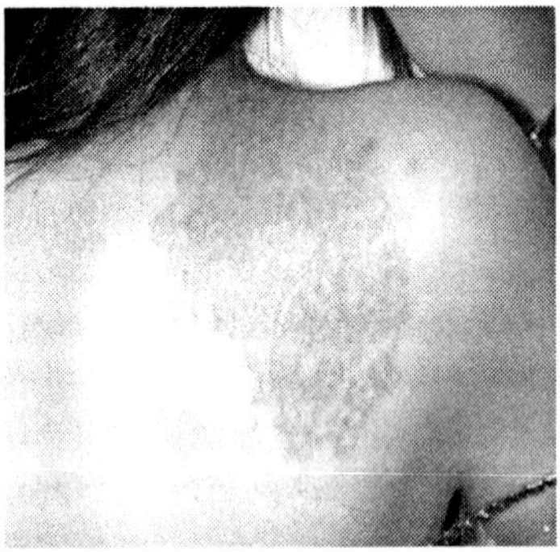

Characteristics of Moles

1. Moles are the most common tumor in humans.

2. Most adults have approximately 15-20 moles.

3. Moles are present in many morphologic types.

4. Moles can transform into a melanoma or malignant Cancer. **(If you suspect a mole may be cancerous, please consult a physician immediately).**

5. Mole recurrence is usually symptomatic of melanoma.
Most moles are benign, but atypical moles (dysplastic nevi) may develop into malignant melanoma, a potentially fatal form of skin cancer. Atypical moles are usually hereditary.

Most atypical moles are bigger than a pencil eraser, and the shape and pigmentation are irregular.

Potentially Cancerous Moles

1. Those with spontaneous ulcerations or bleeding.

2. Those with symptoms such as pain and itching.

3. Congenital and Giant Nevus or Moles.

4. Those showing changes in size and color.

5. Those with unexplained inflammatory changes.

6. Usually occurring in junction and compound moles.

(If you suspect a mole may be cancerous, please consult a physician immediately).

How will I remove them?

The application process is very similar to removing a wart, but it requires specific targeting of the center of the skin mole. You must make sure the mixture is able to penetrate the center of the mole.

Supplies:

The following is a list of things you will need to do the mole removal method:

1. Small Bottle of Castor Oil

Castor oil is widely available at grocery and drug stores. It can also be found online by searching for Castor Oil in any major search engine. There is only one kind of Castor Oil.

2. *Baking Soda (Bicarbonate of Soda)*

Baking soda is widely available at grocery and drug stores.

3. *Sterile Stainless Needle*

Sterile stainless needles are widely available at grocery and drug stores.

4. *Emery Board*

Emery boards are widely available at grocery and drug stores.

5. *Band-aids*

Band-aids are widely available at grocery and drug stores.

The All-Natural Method to Remove Skin Moles:

1. Clean mole(s) with soap and water. Pat dry, but leave the mole(s) damp.

2. Scratch the entire mole's surface with a sterile, stainless needle. Concentrate on the mole's center or base. Use the emery board to scratch and rough up the entire surface of the mole(s). Scratching should be hard enough so that when the mixture is applied, it will penetrate the mole's surface.

3. Mix a teaspoon of Castor Oil with just enough baking soda to make a thin paste, not cake-like or crumbly. If the mixture takes on such a consistency, you will need to add more oil. **A new paste should be used each time you apply the mixture to your mole(s).**

4. Rub a small amount into the mole(s) until it is partially absorbed (this will take approximately 1 or 2 minutes). Make sure you apply enough so the areas you have scratched are covered completely.

5. After the initial application, apply a little more of the mixture over the top and cover with a band-aid.

6. Repeat steps one, three, four, and five, 3 three times a day: Once in the morning, once in the afternoon, and once again right before you go to bed. **You will not have to scratch the surface of the mole after the first time.**

7. Be Patient! It usually takes from 3 days to 3 weeks for the mole(s) to fall out. However, since everyone's body is different, the process may take longer. For this reason keep doing this process until the mole has fallen off completely.

Important Notes:

Scratching is the most important part of the process, since it allows the mixture to penetrate to the core of the mole(s)! If you can't use both hands, you may need another person to help you with that step.

Certain types of mole(s) are very hard. It usually helps to soak them in warm soapy water for 20-30 minutes before scratching. If necessary, simply scratch harder to penetrate the outer layer.

If a slight stinging sensation is not felt, the mixture has not penetrated the mole(s) and the application may not work properly. Scratch deeper and reapply.
Prior to using this method, calluses covering mole(s) should be softened and removed by immersing them in warm to hot water for 15-20 minutes.

Treated mole(s) should be covered at all times when the mixture is applied. Be careful not to disturb or remove the band-aid, because premature removal can slow the healing process.

The mole(s) will usually fall off anywhere between 3 days to 3 weeks, though some individuals taking as long as six weeks.

Redness on the skin around the treated mole(s) is a natural occurrence, and indicates the healing is progressing. Such discoloration quickly disappears.

Pink or red tissue is normal after the mole falls off. Normally, the pinkness fades as the tissue becomes environmentally conditioned. Skin tones normally balance out within 15 days, although some people may require several weeks for skin tones to return to normal.

Precautions:

The castor oil and baking soda mixture is for external use only. If the mixture gets into the eyes, flush thoroughly with water. If unusual discomfort arises, consult a physician.

It worked! What can I do to make sure they don't come back?

Most moles develop from sun exposure. Sun exposure can come from either direct or indirect sunlight. Care should be taken to reduce your sunlight exposure. The following tips can help:

Winter sunlight

Take care to avoid excess sun exposure in the winter. Even though winter sunlight may not seem as harsh as other times of the year, it can be just as damaging as summer sunlight.

Minimize Sun Exposure

Try to plan your outdoor activities around when the sunlight is weaker, before 10:00 am and after 3:00 pm. Sunlight is reflected off of water, snow, sand and concrete. Cloudy or overcast days can still let sunlight through.

Shade

If you have to be outside during peak sunlight hours, try to stay in the shade! Consider using an umbrella if there is no natural shade.

Cover Up

Clothing puts a physical barrier between your skin and the harmful rays of the sun.

Sunscreen

Make sure your sunscreen protects against both UVA and UVB rays and that it has a sun protective factor (SPF) of 30 or more. Reapply frequently, because:

1. It can rub off.
2. Sunlight exposure can decrease a sunscreen's effectiveness.

Although most of the harmful effects of the sun occur during childhood, it is a good idea to be aware of how you can protect yourself from the sun whenever possible.

All About Skin Tags

What are skin tags?

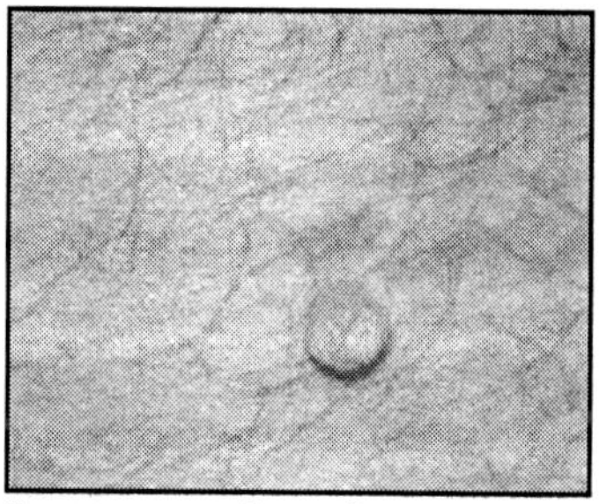

Skin Tags (acrochordons) are small, brown or flesh-colored growths of skin that are typically narrow at their base.
They comprise soft flaps of skin that vary in size from miniscule to the size of a pencil eraser. They do not cause pain unless they become twisted, irritated, or inflamed.

Skin tags are likely to grow on skin surfaces that are hot, moist or frequently rubbed. Skin tags usually appear around the neck, under the arms, under the breasts, in groin creases, and on the inside of the upper thigh. The exact reason skin tags form is not known.

AMA Skin Tag Removal Strategies

Laser Surgery:

The skin tag cells are destroyed by application of a laser.

There can be pain associated with this procedure can be painful, but as with all removal treatments, the pain is generally short-lived and can be mitigated with an over-the-counter painkiller.

The procedure is expensive, however, and may not fit in many patients' budgets.

Extraction:

Skin tags are often removed by incision, either cut off with a scalpel or surgical scissors. The cost of such procedures ranges between $50 and $150.

First, the skin tag area is injected with Lidocaine to numb it. Ironically, this procedure alone is very painful. Then, the skin tag is cut out, often leaving a substantial scar.

Occasionally, the skin tag is also biopsied for cancer.

Electro-Cauterization:

A heated electric wire is applied to the growth and destroys the skin tag. Prices for this procedure vary widely.

Suture:

The skin tag may be removed by wrapping suture around it and cutting off the blood supply. The skin tag usually falls off in about two to three weeks.

This treatment unfortunately leaves the "root" of the skin tag, and it may grow back or leave a raised bump in its place. This also can be a very painful treatment.

The costs associated with suturing can be substantial, and range from $50 to $200. In most cases, you will only be charged the cost of an office call, along with a small amount for the materials used in the procedure.

Cryosurgery or Freezing with Nitrogen:

The skin tag may be frozen with liquid nitrogen, which will require several visits to the doctor's office. Liquid nitrogen is applied directly to the skin tag in order to freeze the growth and destroy the tissue.

This procedure is very painful and in some cases requires an injection of Lidocaine to numb the area before the freezing procedure can begin. The numbing treatment sometime hurts as much as the freezing.

There is also a high risk of scarring with this procedure. Costs range from $50 to $150.

Important Note: Surgical treatments can be painful, may lead to blood loss, and need proper care to reduce the risk of infections during the period of healing.

Disclaimer: This information is not meant to be a substitute for professional medical advice. It is always best to consult with a physician about serious health concerns. This information is in no way intended to diagnose illnesses or offer remedies.

How will I remove them?

The process is very similar to removing a mole, but requires specific targeting of the skin tag "neck" and base area.

Supplies:

The following is a list of things you will need to do the skin tag removal method below:

1. Small Bottle of Castor Oil

Castor oil is widely available at grocery and drug stores. It can also be found online by searching for Castor Oil in any major search engine. There is only one kind of Castor Oil.

2. Baking Soda (Bicarbonate of Soda)

Baking soda is widely available at grocery and drug stores.

3. Sterile Stainless Needle

Sterile stainless needles are widely available at grocery and drug stores.

4. Emery Board

Emery boards are widely available at grocery and drug stores.

5. Band-aids

Band-aids are widely available at grocery and drug stores.

The All-Natural Method to Remove Skin Tags:

1. Clean skin tag(s) with soap and water. Pat dry, but leave the skin tag(s) damp.

2. Scratch the entire skin tag's surface with a sterile, stainless needle. Concentrate on the skin tag's center or base. Use the emery board to scratch and rough up the entire surface of the skin tag(s). Scratching should be hard enough so that when the mixture is applied, it will penetrate the skin tag's surface.

3. Mix a teaspoon of Castor Oil with just enough baking soda to make a thin paste, not cake-like or crumbly. If the mixture takes on such a consistency, you will need to add more oil. **A new paste should be used each time you apply the mixture to your skin tag(s).**

4. Rub a small amount into the skin tag(s) until it is partially absorbed (this will take approximately 1 or 2 minutes). Make sure you apply enough so the areas you have scratched are covered completely.

5. After the initial application, apply a little more of the mixture over the top and cover with a band-aid.

6. Repeat steps one, three, four, and five, 3 three times a day: Once in the morning, once in the afternoon, and once again right before you go to bed. **You will not have to scratch the surface of the skin tag after the first time.**

7. Be Patient! It usually takes from 3 days to 3 weeks for the skin tag(s) to fall out. However, since everyone's body is different, the process may take longer. For this reason keep doing this process until the skin tag has fallen off completely.

Important Notes:

Scratching is the most important part of the process, since it allows the mixture to penetrate to the core of the skin tag(s)! If you can't use both hands, you may need another person to help you with that step.

Certain types of skin tag(s) are very hard. It usually helps to soak them in warm soapy water for 20-30 minutes before scratching. If necessary, simply scratch harder to penetrate the outer layer.

If a slight stinging sensation is not felt, the mixture has not penetrated the skin tag(s) and the application may not work properly. Scratch deeper and reapply.

Treated skin tag(s) should be covered at all times when the mixture is applied. Be careful not to disturb or remove the band-aid, because premature removal can slow the healing process. The skin tag(s) will usually fall off anywhere between 3 days to 3 weeks, though some individuals taking as long as six weeks.

Redness on the skin around the treated skin tag(s) is a natural occurrence, and indicates the healing is progressing. Such discoloration quickly disappears.

Pink or red tissue is normal after the skin tag falls off. Normally, the pinkness fades as the tissue becomes environmentally conditioned. Skin tones normally balance out within 15 days, although some people may require several weeks for skin tones to return to normal.

Precautions:

The castor oil and baking soda mixture is for external use only. If the mixture gets into the eyes, flush thoroughly with water. If unusual discomfort arises, consult a physician.

All About External Genital Warts

(Not to be used for Internal Genital Warts. Please consult a physician.)

What are genital warts?

External Genital Warts are a troubling and depressing problem for both men and women. They are caused by the same virus that causes warts throughout the entire body, HPV (human papilloma virus)

Patients often mistake Genital Warts as a more serious sexually-transmitted disease (STD). Such misunderstanding understandably causes severe anxiety and emotional trauma for sufferers, their sexual partners, and their families.

Although caused by the HPV virus, external genital warts can be highly contagious and spread rapidly around the thighs and genital areas. Immediate steps must be taken to strengthen the immune system against the virus and to destroy the virus before it grows and replicates.

AMA Genital Warts Removal Strategies

Liquid Nitrogen:

Warts on the genitals may be frozen with liquid nitrogen (cryotherapy). The doctor applies the liquid nitrogen over a number of office visits, until the warts are gone. The process can be very painful, given the sensitivity of the affected areas.

Podophyllin:

Your doctor may also treat Warts on the genitals with weekly doses of podophyllin. Your doctor may also put a medicine called podofilox (brand name: Condylox or Aldera) on the warts. The effectiveness rate of these treatments is roughly 55%, not exactly a great chance of success.

Loop Electro-Surgical Excision Procedure (LEEP):

With this method, the doctor passes a sharp instrument shaped like a loop underneath the wart, cutting the wart out of the skin. This process can be very painful, and require 6 months to a year for recovery. The probability for scarring is also high.

CO2 Laser Surgery:

For large warts in the genital area, laser surgery may be needed for complete removal. Although the process is easier on the skin and surrounding areas, the procedure can be expensive.

Interferon Injections:

If genital warts don't go away after they've been treated with the methods described above, your doctor may try an interferon injection into the affected area. Interferon is a chemical made by our bodies, which helps our immune system fight infection. An injection of interferon into the wart may help your body's immune system fight the virus that is causing the wart.

Generally, interferon is injected into warts twice a week for up to 8 weeks, or until the warts are eradicated. This type of procedure is very expensive, with each injection running upwards of $200. This technique is only about 50% effective.

Important Note: Surgical treatments can be painful, may lead to blood loss, and need proper care to reduce the risk of infections during the period of healing.

Disclaimer: This information is not meant to be a substitute for professional medical advice. It is always best to consult with a physician about serious health concerns. This information is in no way intended to diagnose illnesses or offer remedies.

How do I remove them?

For removing genital warts, you will NOT be using the same directions for moles, warts and skin tags, since baking soda will cause a small amount of irritation in the affected area, and you should not use it.

In this procedure, you will only be using the castor oil to remove the warts from your genital area. Unlike the other techniques, you will not be using a sterile stainless needle or an emery board on the affected area.

Supplies:

The following is a list of things you will need to do the genital warts method below:

1. *Small Bottle of Castor Oil*

Castor oil is widely available at local grocery and drug stores. It can also be found online by searching for Castor Oil in any major search engine. There is only one kind of Castor Oil.

2. *Cotton Swabs*

Cotton swabs are widely available at grocery and drug stores.

The All-Natural Method to Remove Genital Warts:

1. Clean the affected area with soap and water. Pat dry until the area is completely dry.

2. Take the bottle of castor oil and squeeze a small amount onto a cotton swab. Gently rub the cotton swab on the affected area, applying generous amounts. DO NOT cover the area with a band-aid.

3. Repeat steps one and two, 3 times a day (morning, afternoon, and evening).

4. Be Patient! It usually takes from 3 days to 3 weeks for the genital wart to disappear. However, since everyone's body is different, the process may take longer. For this reason keep doing this process until the wart has fallen off completely.

Precautions:

Castor oil for genital warts is for external use only. If you have internal genital warts, you will need to consult a physician.

Frequently Asked Questions

Question:

Why do I need to use a band-aid?

Answer:

If you do not use a band-aid to cover the mixture, it will dry up very quickly and become impotent. The mixture works best when moist; using a band-aid maintains the moisture in the mixture for a longer period of time.

This allows the mixture to penetrate the mole, wart or skin tag, and start the removal process. The band-aid also ensures the mixture does not fall off the area.

Question:

Can I follow the steps in the book without using the needle or emery board?

Answer:

No. If you do not complete this step, the mixture will not penetrate deep enough into the mole, wart or skin tag. Again, you are not puncturing the area, but simply scratching it.

Because you are not trying to make yourself bleed, the technique should not hurt. However, it might sting a slightly.

Question:

Do I scratch the area everyday?

Answer:

No. You only scratch the area on the first day and first application.

Question:

What is Castor Oil? Where can I find it?

Answer:

Castor Oil has been used therapeutically in ancient India, China, Persia, Egypt, Africa, Greece, Rome, the Americas, and in 17th-century Europe. Today it is used as an emollient and skin softener. It also is employed in the treatment of gastrointestinal maladies, lacerations, and other skin disorders such as psoriasis. Castor oil is also used to boost your immune system. It is found in many skin care products.

The castor oil should be cold pressed and cold processed, with no hexane.

You can find castor oil in your local supermarket, drug store or health store. You can also purchase castor oil online by following through the following link.

http://www.baar.com

Question:

Is Baking Soda also called Bicarbonate of Soda?

Answer:

Yes. Baking soda is also known as Bicarbonate of Soda.

Question:

I have been using the techniques in the book for 3 days and so far nothing has happened. What should I do?

Answer:

Don't panic! Continue following the steps daily. For most people, the process takes anywhere from 3 days to 3 weeks.

Question:

My mole, wart or skin tag is not drying up and falling off. It is dissolving. Is this normal?

Answer:

Yes. The dissolving of the mole, wart or skin tag occurs in a small percentage of the population. It is completely normal and will not harm your skin.

Continue following the steps in the book until the mole, wart or skin tag has completely disappeared.

Question:

What if my mole, wart or skin tag has not disappeared completely after three weeks? Will these techniques still work?

Answer:

Yes, do not quit! For a small percentage of the population, it takes more than 3 weeks for successful removal. For some it is one month, and for others it is up to two months.

If you have not seen results after two months, then the technique will not work for you. If this is the case, please take advantage of our refund policy.

Question:

I have genital warts. What do I do?

Answer:

Follow the steps in the Genital Warts section. It involves simply using castor oil on the area to get rid of the warts. More details are provided earlier in the book.

Final Thoughts

The more consistent you are with this procedure, the faster your results will arrive. You can bathe and shower normally, since soap will not interfere with the technique. Just remember to reapply the mixture and cover with a band-aid after you have showered.

If you find you are sensitive to the baking soda you may use the Castor Oil alone with the band-aid, and the process will still work; it will just be a little slower in some cases.

When the wart, mole or skin tag falls off, your skin will be scar free and 100% healthy. As stated earlier, in some cases the skin may be somewhat pink, but this discoloration will go away and you will be left with healthy skin.

Removing my moles and warts has greatly enhanced my life. I learned that not all problems could be solved by "consensus reality solutions."

Surgery, drugs and over-the-counter products may have their own negative side effects and don't necessarily affect the origin of the problem. I personally try to maintain my life in balance without them.

This book has related my personal experience about the incredible results I attained during my quest to remove my own moles, warts and skin tags.

"Again, I do not purport to treat or cure any disease. I am simply sharing my personal experience."